weight loss for women 2024

The Ultimate Guide to Successful Weight Loss for Women

SONIA FLETCHER

SONIA FLETCHER

ULTIMATE GUIDE TO WEIGHT LOSS FOR WOMEN

INTRODUCTION — 6

PART I: THE BASICS — 9

- **INTRODUCTION TO WEIGHT LOSS FOR WOMEN** — 9
- **UNDERSTANDING YOUR BODY** — 11
- **SETTING WEIGHT LOSS GOALS** — 14
- **NUTRITION BASICS FOR WEIGHT LOSS** — 16
- **SETTING HEALTHY EATING HABITS** — 19
- **INTERMITTENT FASTING** — 22
- **SLEEP FOR HEALTH AND WELLNESS** — 24
- **STRENGTHENING YOUR MINDSET FOR WEIGHT LOSS** — 26
- **MANAGING STRESS AND ANXIETY** — 28

PART II: MEAL PLANNING AND EXERCISE — 31

- **MEAL PLANNING AND PREP STRATEGIES** — 31
- **SHOPPING FOR HEALTHY FOODS** — 33
- **CALORIE COUNTING 101** — 35

- **CALCULATING YOUR MACROS**   39
- **NUTRITION GOALS FOR WOMEN#**   40
- **UNDERSTANDING INTUITIVE EATING**   44
- **EXERCISES FOR WEIGHT LOSS**   46
- **EXERCISING AT HOME**   48
- **WEIGHT TRAINING FOR WOMEN**   49
- **UNDERSTANDING YOUR ACTIVITY LEVELS**   51

PART III: WEIGHT MAINTENANCE   53

- **EXPLORING DIFFERENT DIETS**   53
- **MAINTAINING A BALANCED DIET**   55
- **MANAGING FOOD CRAVINGS**   57
- **TIME MANAGEMENT TIPS**   58
- **INCORPORATING SUPERFOODS INTO YOUR DIET**   61
- **SETTING ACHIEVABLE GOALS FOR WEIGHT LOSS**   63
- **STAYING MOTIVATED FOR WEIGHT LOSS**   64

- **TIPS FOR STICKING TO YOUR PLAN** — 66

- **AVOIDING WEIGHT LOSS PLATEAUS** — 68

- **INCORPORATING PHYSICAL ACTIVITY INTO EVERYDAY LIFE** — 70

- **MEAL PLANNING FOR BUSY SCHEDULES** — 72

PART IV: LIFESTYLE CHANGES — 74

- **FINDING SOCIAL SUPPORT** — 74

- **MAKING TIME FOR YOURSELF** — 75

- **PREVENTING BINGE EATING** — 78

- **UNDERSTANDING MENTAL HEALTH AND WELLNESS** — 80

- **IMPROVING BODY IMAGE AND SELF-ESTEEM** — 82

- **SETTING LONG-TERM GOALS AND STRATEGIES** — 84

PART V: OTHER CONSIDERATIONS — 86

- **DEALING WITH FOOD ALLERGIES** — 86

- **MANAGING POLYCYSTIC OVARIAN SYNDROME** — 88

- **MANAGING ENDOMETRIOSIS** — 89

- **UNDERSTANDING THYROID DYSFUNCTION** — 92
- **EATING WITH DIABETES** — 94
- **THE AFTERMATH OF WEIGHT LOSS SURGERY** — 95
- **WORKING WITH A DIETICIAN** — 96

CONCLUSION — 98

INTRODUCTION

Elle was once an overweight woman who found her life lacking purpose and joy. She was constantly unhappy, consumed with self-loathing and had entirely given up hope of ever achieving her ideal body image.

One day, through sheer determination and a newfound sense of inner strength, she decided to make a change and start a weight loss journey. It was a decision that helped her tap into her potential and experience a newfound sense of clarity.

Elle started her journey with small steps. She began to cut back on carbohydrates, eliminated sugar and processed foods from her diet. She would focus on eating only healthy plant-based meals to fuel her body. She committed to exercising at least four days a week; combining strength training, yoga, and low-intensity cardio.

As her routine began to become second nature, Elle grew in determination and discipline. She said "no" to late-night snacking, opted for water instead of sugary drinks, and began to appreciate the way her body was transforming.

The journey had its share of obstacles. Elle faced the temptation of junk food and the resulting guilt from not being able to follow through with her plans. But instead of giving up, she used these ideas to further motivate her and create a clear reminder of her end goal.

With each passing month, Elle felt more energy, enthusiasm, and self-love. And when the time came to finally check the scale, she realized she had achieved her goal. She was 30-pounds lighter and had a newfound sense of accomplishment.

Today, Elle is an example of what happens when you stay the course. From rejecting unhealthy habits and recognizing her own worth to running a health and wellness firm, Elle is the woman that she once imagined herself to be. Her transformation helps to remind how powerful determination can be.

Women are under immense pressure to maintain a healthy, attractive figure. There have been waves of "diet culture" over the years and society continues to emphasize beauty standards that focus on thinness. With this widespread obsession with thinness comes health repercussions, both physical and mental, for many women.

This book provides an honest look at the weight loss journey for women. We explore the intersection between body image and mental health, consider the pros and cons of popular diet plans, and provide tangible advice for achieving healthier lifestyle habits. We also tackle the stigma associated with being a "plus size" woman, and offer helpful resources for gaining a positive body image.

Our goal is to empower women to make educated decisions about their diets and health, and to achieve their desired physique in a safe and sustainable way. We want to provide a judgment-free space so that those embarking on the weight loss journey can be honest and true with their thoughts and feelings, while still coming away with lasting results.

SONIA FLETCHER

This book offers valuable information for anyone seeking to gain better self-esteem and long-term fitness. We hope that it encourages readers to have body-positive conversations and to challenge the beauty standards of today that are oftentimes unrealistic and, in some cases, harmful.

We invite you to take this immersive journey with us—let's empower ourselves as women and learn to embrace and celebrate our differences.

SONIA FLETCHER

PART I: THE BASICS

Introduction to Weight Loss for Women

It appears that more and more ladies are making efforts to maintain or get a smaller figure in modern society. Millions of women worldwide aspire to this objective, which is now easier and more effective to achieve than ever. This book strives to give you all the tools and knowledge need to accomplish that goal.

Regardless of your personal objectives, this overview of weight reduction for women can guide you in making the right decisions to maximise your progress towards a healthy body. You can significantly lower your body weight and become in shape in a rather short amount of time with the right commitment and strategy.

You should think about and decide what kind of exercise will best suit your needs before embarking on this new journey. Would you rather work out in a gym or with a fitness group, or do you prefer to work alone?

After deciding on your preferred form of exercise, you should concentrate on diet. If you decide to go down the calorie-reduction route, you should consult a nutritionist or doctor before beginning the diet to get expert guidance on the best course of action.

ULTIMATE GUIDE TO WEIGHT LOSS FOR WOMEN

Success depends on maintaining a balanced diet, and it's crucial to be hydrated and consume adequate fluids throughout the day. Include lots of lean proteins, whole grains, and healthy fats in your meal plan, as well as fresh fruits and vegetables. Your motivation and, more significantly, your energy will be maintained thanks to this base.

Additionally, you must educate yourself on the fundamentals of nutrition and learn how to accurately determine your daily calorie needs. Focusing on making a long-lasting lifestyle change is crucial, and knowing how to estimate your body's nutritional requirements is the ideal starting point.

For weight loss to be successful, exercise is essential. You can opt to focus on quick yet intense HIIT (High Intensity Interval Training) sessions or engage in more calming and moderate-intensity exercises like yoga, depending on your own goals. In order to finish your adventure, keep in mind to start off at a comfortable pace and choose activities that you can easily maintain.

Last but not least, it's critical to adhere to predetermined goals, whether they are focused on exercise, diet, or managing the occasional nutritional lapse. Establishing a system of prizes for each success is another excellent motivator that will keep your sights on the goal as you make the transition to a healthy physique.

You will be astounded by what you may accomplish in a relatively short amount of time by heeding their suggestions and working tirelessly towards your objectives. Although maintaining good health and fitness is difficult, anything is attainable with the appropriate commitment and determination. Good fortune!

SONIA FLETCHER

Understanding Your Body

Understanding your body is the key to unlocking long-term success when it comes to weight loss. Building a reasonable and sustainable weight loss programme that works over time requires understanding how your body functions and reacts to food and physical changes.

This book will offer a thorough examination of the science and physiology of the numerous systems that make up the human body and how they relate to weight management. Learn how to successfully create a tailored, fact-based programme to reach a long-lasting, healthy body weight by reading on to learn about metabolism, diet, exercise, and behaviour change.

Metabolism

Your body employs the metabolic process to convert food into energy. It is influenced by the quantity of food you eat as well as the kinds of everyday activities you partake in. Understanding your personal metabolic rate is crucial to regulating your body weight because no two people have the same metabolism.

The quantity of calories your body must burn each day to maintain your weight is known as your basal metabolic rate (BMR). Your BMR is influenced by a wide range of factors, such as age, gender, body composition, and heredity. Men frequently have a higher BMR than women since they tend to have more muscular mass. Muscle mass has a higher metabolic activity than fat reserve, needing more energy to sustain.

The thermic effect of food (TEF) is the quantity of energy expended during activities other than those required to sustain life, such as walking, jogging, and exercising. TEF accounts for a fraction of your daily calorie expenditure. TEF is typically higher if you exercise frequently and take part in high-energy activities like weightlifting or jogging. Due to the fact that sustaining muscle mass consumes less calories than growing and toning it does, strength training can also raise basal metabolic rate.

Nutrition

To design a weight loss programme that is sustainable, it is essential to comprehend the science behind diet in addition to your BMR and how physical activity affects your energy production. After all, when it comes to losing weight, what you eat accounts for more than half of the issue.

Choosing nutrient-dense, low-calorie foods, managing portion sizes, and ingesting proteins, carbs, and fats are all dietary aspects of good weight management. Every meal should have protein and fibre as well as a healthy balance of the macronutrients protein, carbohydrate, and fat. A balanced diet that includes all of these macronutrients will help you stay satisfied and energised and stop hunger from undermining your weight loss attempts.

Additional advantages of fibre and protein for controlling weight exist. Fibre acts as a form of "filler" in your stomach, prolonging your feeling of fullness and assisting with appetite control. Protein offers the necessary amino acids for muscle growth, and studies have shown that eating more protein makes you feel fuller longer. Consuming protein also speeds up post-workout recovery and aids in maintaining muscle mass.

Exercise

In terms of managing one's weight, exercise is essential. Your success in losing weight can be strongly impacted by the type of activity you perform, as some exercises burn more calories than others. Fortunately, cutting-edge research has made it simpler than ever to customise workouts for individual clients in order to achieve specific weight loss objectives.

Any programme for weight loss based on exercise should start with cardio. Walking, jogging, biking, swimming, and participating in sports are all cardio workouts. Numerous aerobic workouts can be done with little to no equipment indoors or outdoors. They are an excellent technique to enhance daily caloric expenditure and to establish and maintain a strong cardiovascular system.

A thorough weight loss programme should incorporate strength training in addition to cardiovascular exercise. Weights and resistance training can enhance strength and flexibility while also helping tonify and shape muscular tissue. Because muscle requires more calories to maintain than fat does, strength training also aids in maintaining muscle mass, which increases the amount of calories burned while at rest.

Behavior Modification

Your actions have a variety of effects on your weight. A crucial element of long-term weight loss success is knowing how to alter behaviour to develop healthier eating habits. Setting attainable goals and consistently carrying out the commitment to do so fall under this category.

Making a support structure that you can rely on in difficult times is equally crucial. Your support system, which can include friends, family, coworkers, or other gym goers, should offer motivation and hold you accountable as you strive to meet your weight loss objectives.

Additionally, it's critical to adopt mindful eating practises. Stress, boredom, and eating diversions like television can result in unhealthy snacking and increased intake of processed and high-fat meals. Instead, make an effort to eat mindfully and pay attention to how you feel both during and after a meal. By doing this, you can ensure that your body is receiving the proper nutrition it requires to remain healthy.

SONIA FLETCHER

Setting Weight Loss Goals

Many people aim to lose weight in order to improve their health and general well-being. Setting attainable weight loss targets might help you plan out your success and keep you on track. This chapter will cover creating precise goals for weight loss as well as effective goal-setting techniques.

Why Should You Set Weight Loss Goals?

Any successful weight loss programme must include setting specific, attainable targets for weight loss. Goals provide you a destination that helps keep you motivated and on course as you work towards your aims. In addition to giving you measurable benchmarks to work towards, goals can serve as a source of inspiration and motivation. Goals also add an additional element of accountability. When you have goals that you are working towards, you can periodically look back and assess your progress and change your tactics as necessary.

How to Set Weight Loss Goals

It's crucial to keep the following in mind when setting weight loss objectives:

1. Be Realistic: Self-efficacy is enhanced by goals that are realistic. Make sure your objectives are challenging and attainable, but don't aim too high to avoid disappointment.

2. Concentrate on Behaviours: Pay attention to the behaviours that assist you achieve your goals rather than just the number on the scale. This can entail raising your exercise level, tracking your calorie intake, or maintaining a nutritious diet.

3. Establish both short-term and long-term goals. This will help you maintain perspective on the broader picture. Setting short-term objectives is crucial for maintaining your programme. But it's crucial to keep in mind that the weight on the scale might change from day to day, so focusing only on it can be demoralising.

4. Be Specific: Specify your objectives and monitor your development. Instead of just declaring, "I want to lose weight," for instance, set a specific objective such, "I want to lose 10 pounds in the next 6 weeks."

5. Take the Time to Reflect: Keep in mind to consider your advancement. When you accomplish a goal, pause to reflect on your progress and to rejoice. Recognise your missed opportunities, then take a time to alter your strategy and refocus.

The key to accomplishing your weight loss objectives is developing a successful plan and maintaining your motivation as you go. Setting definite, doable goals is a crucial component of this strategy and can keep you on course. Be realistic, concentrate on behaviours, and make both short-term and long-term goals that are precise when setting your goals. Finally, remember to take the time to evaluate your performance, acknowledge your accomplishments, and refocus when necessary.

Nutrition Basics for Weight Loss

Many people have the common objective of losing weight, and any successful weight loss programme must include nutrition. To lose weight and keep it off, one must follow a balanced diet that is low in fat and calories and high in nutrient-dense foods like fruits, vegetables, and whole grains. The fundamentals of nutrition, including macronutrients and micronutrients, as well as how to ensure that you are supplying your body with the proper nutrients to fuel it for weight reduction and general health, are covered in this book.

Macronutrients

The primary nutrients that your body requires in large amounts are called macronutrients. Carbohydrates, proteins, and fats are some of them. All macronutrients are essential for weight loss since they give your body energy.

Your body uses carbohydrates as its primary fuel source. They are present in foods including grains, fruits, and vegetables and can have simple or complicated structural variations. The ideal type of carbohydrates to eat for weight loss are complex ones because they digest slowly and make you feel filled for longer.

Building muscle and other body tissues depends on proteins. Both plant-based foods like beans, nuts, and legumes and animal products like beef and poultry are sources of protein.

Despite not being required nutrients, fats are crucial for optimum health. The two types of fats—saturated and unsaturated—can be found in both animal and plant items. Unsaturated fats are preferable to saturated fats for weight loss since they are healthier.

Micronutrients

Although your body doesn't require a lot of micronutrients for overall health and wellness, they are nevertheless necessary. The vitamins, minerals, and other substances that make up these nutrients. Vitamin A, Vitamin B, Vitamin C, calcium, iron, magnesium, and potassium are a few examples of micronutrients. Consuming foods high in these nutrients can promote weight loss and excellent health.

Eating for Weight Loss

A balanced diet is necessary for weight loss. Make sure every meal contains an adequate amount of all 3 macronutrients (carbohydrates, proteins, and fats). Eat a diet high in unsaturated fats, lean proteins, and complex carbohydrates. Additionally, it's crucial to consume foods that are low in sugar, calories, and saturated fat and high in fibre.

There is no "one size fits all" recommendation when it comes to portion sizes. In general, it's advisable to start with smaller portions and build them up as necessary. You can avoid overeating by eating smaller meals, which can help you feel fuller more quickly.

Any weight loss programme that is successful must include nutrition. Understanding the fundamentals of nutrition, such as macronutrients and micronutrients, as well as how to consume for weight reduction, is crucial. Long-term weight loss success depends on eating a balanced diet of wholesome foods that are high in nutrients like fruits, vegetables, and whole grains yet low in fat and calories.

Setting Healthy Eating Habits

Making appropriate food choices is a crucial component of developing a lifestyle that supports effective weight loss. To make sure that you are consuming meals that will support your body in accomplishing its goals, eating habits need to be periodically reviewed and altered. It takes time, work, and devotion to establish good eating habits, but the effort is ultimately worthwhile.

1. Adhere to a diet strategy that is suitable for you.

It's crucial to take your unique demands and tastes into account when choosing a diet plan. Create a strategy that fits your lifestyle, keeps you interested, and inspires you. Regularly assess your progress and make any corrections.

2. Substitute judiciously.

Your diet can be significantly impacted by substituting harmful foods with better options. For instance, choose fresh fruits or vegetables over processed fizzy drinks or sweets when choosing snacks. Choose whole grains over refined, processed grains when picking your carbohydrates.

3. Consume a range of foods.

Healthy eating includes consuming a balanced diet. Include a wide range of nutrient-rich foods in your diet, including fruits, vegetables, lean meats, and low-fat dairy items. You can achieve your weight loss objectives by limiting your consumption of unhealthy meals like sweets, red meats, and foods with excessive fat and sodium.

4. Eat regularly spaced meals.

Your body's metabolism will be enhanced by spreading out your meals and snacks throughout the day. Eating regularly will also aid in controlling your hunger and preventing overeating.

5. Make sensible objectives.

Setting attainable nutritional objectives that you may actually achieve is crucial. You may actually be less likely to succeed in your weight-loss objectives if your goals are too ambitious or difficult to maintain.

Setting up good eating habits is crucial for achieving weight loss success. Making wise dietary decisions and attainable goals will help you put your health first and position yourself for success. You may quickly change your eating habits and get to your ideal weight with commitment and perseverance.

Vitality of Hydration

One of the most crucial components of any effective weight-loss plan is hydration. The body needs to be properly hydrated in order to perform at its best. The effects of dehydration on the body can include weariness, constipation, gastrointestinal problems, headaches, and mental impairment. Dehydration makes people want to eat more, which can result in weight gain.

Water flushes impurities from the body and aids in the transport of nutrients into cells. It facilitates digestion and can lessen cravings. Additionally, water can lower hunger and assist in regulating body temperature. In essence, getting enough water can help curb hunger and maintain energy levels.

Staying hydrated has many advantages, including lowering fatigue, enhancing cognitive function, and lowering the risk of high blood pressure, heart disease, and stroke. In fact, when people get enough water in their systems, they can cleanse and absorb nutrients more efficiently.

On a fundamental level, being hydrated promotes weight reduction by giving the body the energy it needs to move around, which increases physical activity. Staying hydrated is a great method to promote weight loss attempts because it can increase metabolism and fat burning.

Additionally, since water doesn't include any extra calories, substituting plain water for sugary drinks can lower the overall caloric intake. Additionally, it supports the body's healthy fat-to-muscle ratio, which is necessary for optimum metabolic and physiological performance.

The last advantage of being hydrated is that it promotes weight loss by lowering inflammation. It is believed that inflammation influences obesity by causing metabolic problems and weight gain. Water consumption in large amounts helps reduce inflammation, which in turn can aid in weight loss.

In conclusion, hydration is crucial to any programme for losing weight. Water is crucial for good health and efficient weight loss since it aids in the body's fat burning process and helps to remove toxins from the system. Make sure you are drinking enough water throughout the day if you're trying to lose a few pounds.

Intermittent Fasting

A well-liked weight loss strategy that has gained popularity recently is intermittent fasting. Long stretches without food or with highly restricted eating are followed by frequent, smaller meals. It has been praised for its many health advantages, including weight loss, higher energy, enhanced cardiovascular health, and improved mental clarity.

Intermittent fasting is not a novel idea; it has long been a feature of numerous religious rituals. However, it has become more well-liked in the modern diet as an intermittent lifestyle approach to weight loss. It has long been a staple of the traditional diets of many nations and religions, including the Ramadan fast in Islam.

By switching your body's energy source from carbohydrates to fat, intermittent fasting causes a switch from quickly and easily burning carbohydrates to more slowly burning fats. During the fasting periods, the body burns off the stored sugar and fat for energy, lowering the body's overall fat level in the process.

Due to the variety of fasting lifestyles available, intermittent fasting is typically easier to sustain than other diets. Simply eating intermittently for certain amounts of time will suffice; there is no need for calorie counting, measuring, or meal plans.

Studies on the health advantages of intermittent fasting have shown that it can lower blood triglyceride and cholesterol levels, control blood sugar levels, reduce inflammation, and slow the ageing process. Furthermore, research indicates that intermittent fasting can aid in weight loss, with some people losing up to 10% of their body weight when fasting. Even the fasting period itself has some advantages. According to studies, thin people who fast on occasion perform better on mental health exams than persons who don't fast.

Depending on how it's done, intermittent fasting can be a secure and efficient method of weight loss. You should carefully plan out your fasting to guarantee safety and maximise health advantages. Select a plan that fits your needs in terms of duration, and include a supplemental nutrition plan outlining your health goals both before and after the fast. Processed foods should be avoided when fasting as they provide very little to no nutritional value to the body. Additionally, since some diets may make you feel weak or dizzy, it's crucial to pay attention to your hunger cues. Additionally, it's crucial to make sure you're getting enough fluids, vitamins, and minerals to make up for the fluids you lose when fasting.

If done correctly, intermittent fasting can be a successful weight-loss strategy. It might also have some intriguing health advantages. Before starting an intermittent fasting regimen, like with any diet, it is crucial to speak with your doctor to be sure it is the right course of action for you. Intermittent fasting can result in healthy, successful weight loss as well as increased mental and physical health with the correct preparation and execution.

Sleep for Health and Wellness

The quality of your sleep has a big impact on your wellbeing. How well and how much you sleep has a big impact on how you feel and how you behave physically and emotionally. Your body's capacity to control hormones and hunger is compromised by poor or insufficient sleep, which contributes to weight gain. On the other hand, maintaining a healthy weight and lowering your chance of developing certain disorders linked to being overweight are both benefits of getting enough good sleep.

Getting enough restful sleep also encourages physical activity by boosting energy levels and reducing weariness. Inflammation can weaken the immune system, increase the risk of disease, and contribute to maintaining a healthy weight. Good sleep also helps to reduce inflammation.

Mentally, getting enough sleep is crucial for controlling your mood, managing your stress, and sharpening your focus. Our ability to think creatively and digest new information is aided by sleep. Our bodies are unable to digest information when we don't get enough sleep, which also affects our capacity to focus and maintain attention.

You can take the following actions to get improved quality and quantity of sleep:

Maintain proper sleep hygiene by creating routines and habits that will help you unwind and fall asleep. The bedroom should be cold and dark. At least an hour before going to bed, turn off any screens (TV, computer, smartphone).

Limit caffeine consumption: Give your body plenty of time to unwind and rest by avoiding coffee six to eight hours before bed.

Regular exercise has been demonstrated to enhance the quality of sleep and to help reduce stress.

It is best to avoid eating after midnight because it may disrupt the hormones that regulate appetite and make it hard to fall or remain asleep.

Getting adequate rest can ensure that all of your hard work pays off, regardless of the diet and exercise programme you're following as part of your overall weight reduction and health journey. You can attain your objective of health and wellness and manage your weight by eating a balanced diet, exercising frequently, and getting plenty of sleep.

Strengthening Your Mindset for Weight Loss

Many individuals focus on the physical side of things, such as going to the gym and eating well, when it comes to losing weight. While this is unquestionably vital, addressing the mental side of achieving a healthy weight is frequently necessary to ensure long-term weight loss success. In order to achieve your weight loss goals and keep them over the long run, you must strengthen your attitude.

Realising that weight loss is a journey and not a destination is the first step in developing a more positive outlook. It requires commitment and dedication to reach your target weight and keep it off. You must have confidence in your ability to complete the task at hand and in the eventual success of your endeavours. You also need to develop the ability to maintain consistency in your efforts and discover drive to press on even in the face of setbacks.

The next step is to develop an optimistic outlook. An optimistic outlook is necessary for a successful weight loss journey. Consider it a chance to enhance your health and wellbeing rather than a challenge. Focus on your accomplishments and be grateful for the progress you achieve rather than the challenges you confront. Also, think on the good things that will happen in your life as a result of losing weight.

Finding the underlying fundamental reasons of your bad eating patterns is the next step. Sometimes, negative eating habits can result from specific mental or emotional behaviours. Because of this, it's critical to investigate the root causes of these patterns and find a healthy, effective strategy to deal with them.

The fourth step is to prioritise your own well-being. Regular self-care is essential for maintaining your physical and emotional health. Invest in relaxing and physically empowering activities like yoga, massages, and a balanced diet. Be sure to get enough sleep every night, and look for ways to lessen stress in your life.

Having a plan and following it is the fifth and last phase. You should make an action plan for yourself and make a commitment to following it once you have developed a good mindset and determined the causes of your unhealthy eating behaviours. Keep track of your development as you go along and make constant modifications to make sure you stay on course.

Strengthening your mindset for effective weight loss is made much easier by following these strategies. You'll be able to maintain your motivation, recognise your accomplishments, and remain dedicated to achieving your goals. As a result, you'll be able to maintain your concentration and weight management as you make the transition to a healthier and happier life.

Managing Stress and Anxiety

Losing weight may be a very challenging and stressful process. Many people who are trying to lose weight deal with a variety of mental and physical effects. Two of the most prevalent emotions that many people go through during the procedure are stress and anxiety. While it's critical to acknowledge these feelings and deal with them in a healthy way, it's also crucial to know how to deal with stress and anxiety to avoid having a detrimental effect on your ability to lose weight.

Creating a good balance between mind and body is one of the most crucial steps in managing stress and anxiety. This entails maintaining a regular exercise routine and consuming a healthy diet. Exercise releases hormones that function as mood enhancers naturally and helps to lessen the physical impacts of stress and anxiety. Additionally, it's critical to refrain from bad practises including crash diets and supplement use as well as missing meals. Eating the correct mixture of complete, healthy foods will satisfy your hunger and give you the nutrition you need to lose weight successfully.

It's crucial to take the time to unwind and put one's health first in addition to obtaining a balanced state of mind and body. Finding a leisure-focused activity or interest, like yoga, meditation, gardening, or even journaling, can be quite useful. Connecting with nature, whether through hobbies or home decor, is another powerful method for lowering stress and anxiety. Spending time with friends and family, discussing life goals and desires, and organising the steps to take to attain them can all aid in rerouting the mind to produce more favourable results.

SONIA FLETCHER

Last but not least, it's critical to make sure that someone is receiving enough good sleep. According to research, sleep deprivation not only has negative health impacts but also raises stress and anxiety levels. Setting up a regular sleep schedule can be helpful, and relaxing the mind before bed by reading a book or engaging in a mindfulness exercise can assist to reduce tension and worrisome thoughts.

An individual can control their stress and anxiety and avoid any negative effects on their weight reduction efforts by making a conscious effort to pay attention to both their physical and mental wellbeing. People may continue to put in the necessary effort to reach their goals by maintaining a balanced state of mind and body, engaging in activities that help them unwind and reduce stress, and getting enough sleep.

ULTIMATE GUIDE TO WEIGHT LOSS FOR WOMEN

SONIA FLETCHER

PART II: MEAL PLANNING AND EXERCISE

Meal Planning and Prep Strategies

Any effective weight loss plan must include meal planning and preparation techniques. Planning and preparing meals guarantee that the proper foods are eaten at the right times and in the right amounts. Making ensuring that meals adhere to the permitted calorie limits outlined by the diet plan also helps. Since meals are portioned out and saved for later, preparing meals in advance also saves time and helps people avoid overeating.

Choosing a nutritional profile that best meets your individual dietary demands is the first step in meal planning and preparation. Based on dietary limitations, lifestyle, body composition, and exercise levels, different people may have varied dietary demands. To lose weight successfully and sustainably, it's critical to understand exactly what your body requires.

It's time to choose a meal plan once you have a general understanding of your nutritional requirements. There are numerous eating techniques that can be used. While some people choose to concentrate on certain foods, others concentrate on foods arranged by day. Some people opt for online programmes that offer meal plans that are specifically tailored to meet their needs. Meal plans are already included in the majority of weight loss programmes, though some may need further customisation based on personal preferences.

The next stage is to begin meal preparation after selecting a meal plan. Meal preparation takes meal planning and organises it. Meals that are prepared in bulk for later use serve to reduce wastage of time and resources while also limiting overeating. Additionally, it aids in ensuring the nutritional balance of meals. When a meal is actually needed, having meals prepared in advance also saves time. You can save time at mealtime by having prepared meals in the fridge or freezer rather than having to start from scratch.

Making the most of nutrient-dense foods is one of the most crucial meal-prepping advices. Ideal options include protein sources, nutritious carbohydrates, and fresh veggies. The body will be able to obtain the nutrients it requires from these nutrient-dense foods without consuming an excess of empty calories.

Although meal preparation and planning initially require more time and effort, the benefits are great. It saves time, discourages overeating, and guarantees that the body receives all the nutrients required for effective and sustained weight loss. Anyone who wants to achieve and maintain their health and fitness goals should give it a try.

Shopping for Healthy Foods

If you want to lose weight, you must shop for healthy foods. Today, we have a wide range of options at our disposal, some of which are healthy and others which are not. Knowing which foods are not only healthy for you but also aid in weight loss is crucial in light of this. Once you are aware of these foods, you can start making decisions that will help you stay on track with your weight loss objectives.

When choosing nutritious foods, portion control is among the most crucial considerations. When it comes to food, many of us have a tendency to overbuy, which can result in consuming excessive amounts of harmful foods or unhealthy snacks. Pay attention to your purchases and make sure you only make those you truly need. Pre-packaged meals and snacks are frequently found to be useful for regulating portion sizes. These are available online or in wholesome food stores.

It's crucial to opt for locally grown, organic produce wherever you can when purchasing fresh produce. This indicates that the fruits and vegetables you purchase were cultivated in an area that complies with environmental safety regulations. Additionally, this guarantees that the goods you are purchasing have not come into contact with pesticides or other toxins.

What kind of cooking technique you employ is a further factor to take into account when buying nutritious foods. You might wish to swap out some components for healthy ones if you want to lower your cholesterol or fat intake. Olive oil or coconut oil, for instance, can be used as a healthy substitute for butter and margarine.

Prior to purchasing, make sure to review the ingredient list of the product. Despite having a "low fat" or "no sugar added" label, some foods may nevertheless include dangerous additives such artificial sweeteners or trans fats. It's crucial to study the label to confirm if a product described as healthy is actually aiding you in achieving your objectives.

Last but not least, make sure your diet is varied. Eating the same things repeatedly can get dull and discourage you from losing weight since your body loves variety. Make an effort to buy a range of goods to keep things exciting and healthy.

Shopping for healthy foods for weight loss doesn't have to be difficult. If you take your time and research your options, you can find delicious, nutritious options that will help you on your journey to healthier living.

Calorie Counting 101

Although calorie counting can appear difficult, time-consuming, or even daunting, it is a fantastic tool for weight loss and leading a better lifestyle. To help you get started on the road to effective weight loss in the midst of the wealth of nutrition and health information available today, we've put up this Calorie Counting 101 guide.

What Are Calories?

Energy is measured in calories. It is the energy required to increase a gramme of water's temperature by one degree Celsius. It is also the quantity of energy required to maintain our lives and power our bodies. The body utilises calories, which we obtain from the food and beverages we consume, to perform nearly all of its functions, including walking, running, and thinking. We gain weight when we consume more calories than our bodies require, and we lose weight when we consume insufficient calories.

What Is Calorie Counting?

The act of keeping track of your daily calorie intake is known as calorie counting. This assists you in staying inside the daily calorie range that is advised, which may be utilised to manage your weight and even assist you in achieving your fitness and health goals.

Calorie counting can be done informally by keeping a food journal and keeping track of everything you consume. But more thorough tracking is strongly advised if you're serious about achieving your objectives. Accurate and reliable tracking are essential, whether you track manually with paper and a pen or digitally using a tracking programme. Try to measure and weigh your food. This eliminates any uncertainty and guarantees precision for efficient tracking.

How to Count Calories

Learning the fundamentals of nutrition labels is the first step in the calorie counting process. You can typically find the calories on any food or drink item as "Calories per serving." This represents the overall caloric content of one serving of that food. The total number of calories obtained from fat in that dish is shown by the phrase "Calories from fat," which you may also observe.

The first step in the calorie tracking process is understanding the basics of nutrition labels. The number of calories in any food or beverage item is often indicated as "Calories per serving." This shows how many calories are in a serving of that meal overall. You may also see the term "Calories from fat," which indicates the total number of calories gained from fat in particular dish.

Calorie Counting Benefits

Beyond only helping you lose weight, tracking calories can help you understand your body's needs for macro- and micronutrients as well as the consequences of the foods you eat on your energy and general health.

Calorie counting can assist you in maintaining awareness, striking a balance between overeating and undereating, and comprehending the nutritional value (or lack thereof) of various foods in your diet. Planning ahead also involves keeping track of how many calories you consume each day. Understanding the nutritional content of food helps you become more aware of your own demands and preferences.

Calorie counting is an effective weight management technique, but like with any weight loss strategy, always seek out individualised guidance and suggestions from a licenced dietitian or physician. You'll be well on your way to accomplishing your health and wellness objectives if you use Calorie Counting as your guide.

Low-Calorie Alternatives to Regular Foods

As they typically have fewer calories and less fat than traditional foods while occasionally being just as tasty, low-calorie substitutes for familiar foods can be a terrific approach to aid in weight loss. Consuming low-calorie items can help you reduce your overall calorie consumption and keep track of how much you are eating each meal.

The most crucial meal of the day is breakfast, and there are several low-calorie substitutions you can make that won't seem like a sacrifice. Choose a smoothie over sugary cereal. A quick and nutritious smoothie can be made with a banana, almond milk, oats, and a scoop of your preferred protein powder. Alternately, substitute a boiled egg and a small side of seed-based bread with a tablespoon of avocado for the traditional bacon and eggs.

Consider substituting soup for your lunch if you want to reduce your calorie intake. Pick broth-based soups and add veggies like kale, spinach, and mushrooms that are high in nutrients. A vegetarian wrap makes a fantastic low-calorie supper. Grilled or roasted veggies, hummus, and fresh herbs should all be placed inside a lettuce wrap.

You should eat small meals and snacks throughout the day to stay energised and prevent hunger from taking control. In the long run, nuts, seeds, and fresh fruit like berries can be a terrific way to acquire the nourishment you need while also keeping you on track.

Another crucial meal to keep an eye out for while trying to stick to a low-calorie diet is dinner. You can make a lot of low-calorie substitutions and still have a delicious dinner. Consider substituting roasted squash or cauliflower rice for white rice. Choose whole wheat or vegetable-based pasta when making pasta. And if you're in the mood for some beef, choose a substitute like bison or buffalo meat, which is typically thinner than most.

Another crucial meal to keep an eye out for while trying to stick to a low-calorie diet is dinner. You can make a lot of low-calorie substitutions and still have a delicious dinner. Consider substituting roasted squash or cauliflower rice for white rice. Choose whole wheat or vegetable-based pasta when making pasta. And if you're in the mood for some beef, choose a substitute like bison or buffalo meat, which is typically thinner than most.

Calculating Your Macros

It's crucial to calculate your macros if you want to lose weight. The nutrients you need to survive, such as carbs, protein, and fat, are known as macronutrients. It's important to comprehend your individual macronutrient requirements if you want to lose weight. You primarily require three macronutrients: carbs, proteins, and fat.

Your body uses carbohydrates as its primary fuel source, giving you the vigour to carry out your everyday tasks. For the average person, the daily required carbohydrate consumption is about 130 grammes. By multiplying your daily calorie consumption by 0.45, you may determine how many carbohydrates you require. The number of calories per gramme of carbohydrates is 4, therefore if you consume 1,600 calories daily, divide that amount by 4 to get 400 calories. An average day's worth of 400 calories is equivalent to 90 grammes of carbohydrates.

Your body gets the critical amino acids it needs from proteins to function properly. Protein is also known to aid in muscle rehabilitation and tissue repair after exercise. One gramme of protein for every pound of body weight per day is advised. For instance, if you weigh 150 pounds, your daily requirements for protein would be 150 grammes.

The most energy-dense macronutrient is fat, which also gives your body vital fatty acids. Additionally, dietary fat is crucial for hormone synthesis and control. Adults should consume 20% to 35% of their total daily caloric intake as fat, on average. Take your total calorie consumption and multiply it by 0.25 and 0.35 to determine your daily fat intake. Using the previous example as a guide, you would require 40–56 grammes of fat per day to satisfy your needs if you consumed 1,600 calories daily.

The most energy-dense macronutrient is fat, which also gives your body vital fatty acids. Additionally, dietary fat is crucial for hormone synthesis and control. Adults should consume 20% to 35% of their total daily caloric intake as fat, on average. Take your total calorie consumption and multiply it by 0.25 and 0.35 to determine your daily fat intake. Using the previous example as a guide, you would require 40–56 grammes of fat per day to satisfy your needs if you consumed 1,600 calories daily.

Nutrition Goals for Women

Any programme for losing weight that is successful must focus on nutrition. When attempting to lose weight, women in particular should be conscious of their dietary requirements. These are some crucial nutrition objectives for women:

1. Balance Macros: Women should keep track of their intake of macronutrients such protein, carbs, and fats. Women can encourage muscle growth and maintain a healthy weight by eating a variety of these macronutrients.

2. Eat more fruits and veggies: Fruits and vegetables are a good source of fibre, vitamins, and minerals. They are excellent for weight loss because they have less calories. At least five servings of fruits and vegetables per day are recommended for women.

3. Cut Back on Sugar: Added sugars are almost always bad for you and can make you gain weight. Women should try to limit their intake of added sugars and instead concentrate on naturally occurring sugars found in wholesome meals like fruits and vegetables.

4. Opt for Healthy Fats: Consuming healthy fats like those found in avocado, olive oil, and almonds can aid in weight loss. Healthy fats can also aid with desire control and are good for the heart.

5. Increase Fibre Intake: Fibre has various advantages, including assisting in digestion and helping to control blood sugar levels. By consuming high-fiber foods such beans, lentils, whole grains, nuts, and seeds, women should aim to consume 25 to 35 grammes of fibre each day.

6. Drink Lots of Water: Water keeps you hydrated and is necessary for proper body operation. Every day, women should consume at least eight glasses of water.

7. Limit Alcohol Consumption: Alcohol frequently has high calorie and sugar content and might cause weight gain. It is advised that women consume no more than one standard drink per day of alcohol.

Women can achieve their weight loss objectives and enhance their general health by adhering to these seven nutritional objectives. Never forget to get medical advice or speak with a certified nutritionist before making any significant dietary or lifestyle changes.

Establishing Meal Routines

Any effective weight-loss regimen should include establishing regular mealtime routines. Your body's metabolism will stay in check if you eat regular meals and snacks, and you'll be less prone to overeat or select unhealthy snacks. Making healthy decisions is simpler when you have a plan and consistently follow it.

Create a timetable that works with your lifestyle before you begin your meal regimen, taking into account when you'll have time for food preparation, when you can have meals with family, and when you'll have time for snacks. Realising what works for you will help you create a plan that fits your lifestyle.

Breakfast should be consumed every day. Going too long without eating will slow down your metabolism and make losing weight nearly hard. To start your metabolism going, nutritionists advise eating within an hour of waking up each day.

Along with eating regularly throughout the day, it's vital to avoid going more than four to five hours without eating. When people consistently eat snacks in between meals, they are frequently astonished at how quickly hunger may be controlled. Regular snacking will help you control your hunger and make choosing the right portion sizes for meals simpler.

Plan your meals and snacks the previous day to guarantee consistent mealtime habits. You'll be able to stay on track during the week and find it easier to avoid unhealthy snacks if you set out an extra 15 minutes on Sunday to plan your meals for the next week.

Additionally, you need to be aware of the times you eat your meals and snacks. Eating at roughly the same times every day can help you feel more in control of your food choices since it provides you a sense of consistency.

It is crucial to create a regular eating schedule if you want to be successful with your weight loss. The greatest place to start is to create a plan in advance. As you advance, you could discover that adjustments to your routine are required because of travel or busy periods. If this gets too challenging, getting assistance can be a good idea. Ideally, you will be able to properly follow your meal schedule and achieve your weight-loss goal as you grow accustomed to meal times and the things you're eating.

SONIA FLETCHER

Understanding Intuitive Eating

Recognising Intuitive The idea of eating has become more and more well-liked among people who are trying to lose weight. It is a method of eating that places a strong emphasis on the value of paying attention to your body's physical and emotional cues while selecting foods. Instead of adhering to rigorous diet rules or recommendations, the idea is to eat in accordance with your body's demands.

The foundation of intuitive eating is the idea that every person has specific needs, and that their bodies are the greatest experts on what foods to eat and when. This adaptable method of eating entails paying attention to and respecting your individual sensations of hunger and fullness.

Before making any meal decisions, intuitive eating encourages you to consider your feelings and your needs. Instead of feeling bad by forcing yourself to restrict your eating, this internal conversation enables you to choose foods based on what your body is telling you.

Intuitive eating is not substitute for healthy eating or involve denying yourself of the things you enjoy. In contrast, it promotes adaptability and daily attention to your body's demands.

Also appreciating the joy that food can provide is intuitive eating. A natural and balanced diet can include eating enjoyable items as long as they are eaten in moderation. Additionally, it encourages diners to take their time and enjoy each bite, which can lessen the likelihood of overeating.

Developing a compassionate relationship with food and with oneself is crucial to intuitive eating. This is being conscious of how you communicate to yourself about eating and letting go of any associated shame. There is no one size fits all approach to nutrition; every dietary choice is a personal one.

Dementia promotes the weight reduction strategy known as intuitive eating, which involves paying attention to your internal hunger and fullness cues, mindfully satiating any nutritional desires, and lowering any related shame. Although losing weight can be challenging, you can learn to eat in a way that is satisfying and meets your individual needs by adopting the Intuitive Eating method.

Exercises for Weight Loss

A healthy lifestyle includes losing weight, and there are numerous workouts that can assist you in doing so. Your physical and mental health, as well as your general quality of life, can all benefit from exercise.

Finding the ideal diet and exercise regimen for you is the secret to weight loss success. Exercises that increase your heart rate, like jogging, riding, swimming, or walking, help you burn calories and shed pounds. According to research, these activities can lower cholesterol, enhance lean muscle mass, reduce body fat, improve mental health, and even cut the risk of developing diseases like diabetes and heart disease.

Another crucial component of exercise for weight loss is strength training. According to studies, adding strength training to your programme can help you reduce fat and build lean muscle. Gaining muscle through weight exercise increases your ability to burn calories. Additionally, it aids in muscle growth and toning, improving your body's overall appearance and shape.

Another excellent form of exercise for shedding pounds is yoga. According to studies, practising yoga frequently enhances flexibility, balance, and posture. Additionally, yoga improves the body's capacity for relaxation and respiratory control while assisting in stress reduction. This prevents hunger and encourages healthy eating practises. Additionally, it aids in extending the body's range of motion, enhancing overall strength and stamina.

And lastly, interval training is a fantastic weight-loss activity. This form of exercise helps you burn more calories in less time, according to studies. You alternate brief bursts of vigorous activity with periods of less vigorous, or resting, activity during intervals. You can achieve your weight loss objectives by increasing the overall number of calories you burn by increasing the intensity of the activity throughout the intervals.

A crucial component of weight loss is exercise. Exercise can assist you in safely and efficiently achieving your weight loss goals when combined with a balanced diet. A fantastic way to begin your journey to a better living is to incorporate interval training, yoga, strength training, and cardiovascular exercises into your daily routine.

No matter the form of exercise you select, it's crucial to take care of yourself and pay attention to your body. Before starting any fitness programme, be sure to consult your doctor. Start out slowly and increase your intensity and length as your body gets used to the action. You will quickly be on the road to achieving your desired weight loss goals with the proper dietary and activity regimen.

Exercising at Home

An excellent approach to acquire the exercise required for a healthy lifestyle and weight loss is by exercising at home. It might be challenging to commit to going to the gym or playing sports when one has a busy lifestyle. Constructing a home gym inside your own walls is practical.

The first step in setting up a home gym can be to find the equipment that works for you financially. Weights, a yoga mat, possibly a dumbbell rack or a pilates machine, and other essential pieces of equipment can provide you with a variety of activities to select from. Regular walks or jogs, which are arguably the most fundamental and necessary kind of exercise, can be a terrific method to burn calories and get the many health advantages of beginning an exercise regimen.

Setting out a specific time of day for exercise can be a crucial first step in developing a reliable programme. It is advisable to arrange specific days for weight training with the various pieces of home gym equipment and dedicate them to your fitness goals.

Exercises don't always require tools and weights. Simple body weight workouts that may be performed at home include squats, burpees, jumping jacks, and push-ups. Without a lot of equipment, Pilates may be a terrific exercise for toning and strengthening. Without additional equipment, you can easily perform other hobbies at home, including yoga or dancing.

It's useful to keep track of your progress in order to stay motivated to exercise. A wonderful strategy to stay on track is to set short-term, attainable goals and actions. To track repetitions, successes, or advancements in terms of weight loss or circumference loss, keep a fitness notebook. An excellent visual tool to aid in maintaining commitment to a fitness practise is a daily record or journal.

If one commits to an exercise plan, exercising at home can be a terrific method to burn calories and lose weight. Setting up a home gym and selecting the appropriate activities for your fitness budget can help with weight reduction and overall wellness. Anyone may start an exercise routine from within their own four walls given enough time, effort, and commitment.

Weight Training for Women

Women's weightlifting has grown in popularity recently, and for good cause. Women can benefit from weight training in numerous ways, including enhanced strength and endurance, a faster metabolism, and better posture. Weight lifting can also play a significant role in many women's weight loss plans.

Many women find lifting weights scary, but this does not have to be the case. For injury prevention and optimum exercise results, learning good form and technique is crucial. You can get started with a training programme that is customised to your fitness objectives and unique needs with the assistance of a qualified personal trainer or other fitness expert.

The secret to utilising weights to reduce weight is to concentrate on compound workouts that simultaneously target several muscle groups. Squats, bench presses, deadlifts, as well as pull-ups and push-ups, are examples of compound exercises. It's also crucial to use progressive overload, which is gradually raising the resistance as your muscles get used to the exercise.

Along with compound exercises, including certain isolation exercises will assist increase strength and focus on specific body parts that may require more attention. Bicep curls, tricep extensions, and shoulder presses are a few examples of isolation exercises.

Workouts that are circuit-styled are a terrific place for ladies who have never lifted weights before to start. These exercises include alternating between them while taking just brief breaks. This kind of exercise programme has the additional benefit of increasing calorie burn while also assisting in strength development. Additionally, they require little to no equipment, making circuit-style workouts a practical choice for women trying to lose weight.

SONIA FLETCHER

For women seeking to reduce weight, walks, runs, bike rides, and swimming are all excellent exercises that go well with weight training. You can boost your strength and burn more calories by include weight-bearing exercises in your fitness programme while still working towards your weight loss objectives.

Women who wish to get stronger, lose weight, and enhance their general health may consider weight training. You may achieve your fitness and weight loss objectives in a safe and efficient manner with a little bit of knowledge and direction.

Understanding Your Activity Levels

It's crucial to comprehend your exercise levels if you want to lose weight. It's critical to comprehend how your body functions and how to incorporate physical activity into your daily life if you're trying to reduce weight.

To start, it's crucial to understand your resting metabolic rate (RMR). When you are not moving around, your body burns calories at this pace. You may calculate how many calories you must consume each day to maintain your present weight by knowing this figure. It's also critical to be conscious of any persistent pains in your body that appear after engaging in physical activity. Even though you experience discomfort, it's crucial to understand what you can and cannot do.

Second, controlling your weight can be done with knowledge of your exercise levels. Weight and activity levels are negatively correlated: higher activity levels result in lower weight, whereas lower activity levels result in higher weight. In order for your general activity levels to be maintained throughout time, it is crucial to learn how to increase them. This can entail adding particular activities to your weekly routine, such taking a walk or a swim or signing up for a fitness class.

Third, you may manage the meals you eat by being aware of and in charge of your activity levels. The body burns more calories as a result of regular physical activity because it expends more energy. If you're extremely dedicated, you could even use this to replace meals or justify occasional treats. Increasing your exercise level will certainly assist you in achieving your intended weight loss goal in either scenario.

Finally, it's critical to comprehend the effects of insufficient exercise on your body. Insufficient exercise causes a decline in resting metabolic rate, muscle loss, and physical performance. These consequently result in weight gain and a general deterioration of physical health. In order to achieve better weight loss results, it is crucial to engage in regular physical exercise and form healthy eating habits.

In conclusion, it's crucial to comprehend your activity levels if you want to lose weight. To define and manage your activity levels, it's crucial to understand your resting metabolic rate and establish a regular physical activity schedule. Additionally, raising your activity level continuously will maximise the amount of weight you can lose over a given time frame. Regular exercise is important for overall health and wellbeing as well as for decreasing weight.

PART III: WEIGHT MAINTENANCE

Exploring Different Diets

Investigating various diets can be a very useful strategy for weight loss. Your chances of success can be considerably increased by selecting the diet that is best for your unique demands and way of life. Even though certain diets drastically cut your caloric intake and speed up weight reduction, these kinds of diets might not be long-term maintainable. Other diets emphasise consuming the proper ratio of macro- and micronutrients so that your body will have the energy it needs to continue losing weight.

Researching diets should include comparing them based on convenience, affordability, and sustainability. There are many different diets to consider, and each one has its own advantages, disadvantages, and guidelines. Consider the following common diets to help you reach your weight loss objectives:

Diet known as the "keto" is high in fat, moderate in protein, and low in carbohydrates. Your body must enter a metabolic condition known as ketosis in order to start burning fat for energy instead of carbohydrates. This kind of diet can be helpful because it helps to control hunger hormones and decrease appetite.

Mediterranean Diet: This diet is based on plants and emphasises lean proteins, healthy fats, and whole-grain carbohydrates. Your risk of getting chronic diseases can be lowered by consuming a wide variety of plant-based foods.

An eating pattern known as intermittent fasting alternates between periods of eating and fasting. By allowing your body to rest, this kind of diet can help you maintain healthy blood sugar levels.

Low-Fat Diet: This is a diet that places a focus on low-fat meals and restricts trans and saturated fats. Limiting your intake of fat can help you lose weight, manage your cholesterol levels, and lower your chance of getting certain diseases.

Paleo diet: The Paleo diet places an emphasis on eating full, unprocessed foods such fruits, vegetables, nuts, and healthy fats. Consuming whole foods can assist to promote gut health and reduce inflammation.

Whole Foods Plant-Based Diet: This eating style places an emphasis on unprocessed plant foods such whole grains, legumes, and vegetables. Consuming whole foods can help you stay healthier overall and lower your risk of developing chronic diseases.

Diet that places an emphasis on high-protein, high-fat, and healthy fats is called the Atkins diet. This diet can manage hunger hormones and decrease appetite.

No matter what kind of diet you choose, it's crucial to make sure you're consuming the correct number of calories and obtaining all the nutrients you need for good health. Any good weight loss regimen should have proper nutrition as its foundation. While experimenting with various diets can be a terrific approach to start losing weight, it's crucial to do so in a way that supports your unique requirements and objectives. For any diet plan to be successful, eating a wide range of healthful foods and paying attention to portion control are vital.

Maintaining a Balanced Diet

To reach and keep a healthy weight, one must follow a balanced diet. High-quality proteins, complex carbs, healthy fats, vitamins, minerals, and water make up a diet that is well-balanced. A balanced diet can help you get the nutrients your body needs to lose weight and keep it working at its best.

Proteins

Every meal should contain proteins from lean meats, fish, dairy, legumes, nuts, and seeds. Proteins are crucial nutrients that support energy production and muscle growth and repair. Eating enough protein will help you feel filled for longer and lose weight because it requires more energy to digest than other foods.

Complex Carbohydrates

A variety of necessary vitamins and minerals are provided by the complex carbohydrates found in vegetables, wholegrain breads, legumes, and whole grains. A healthy diet should be built around these complex carbs. Due to their slow digestion, they reduce blood sugar surges and prolong energy levels.

Good Fats

A balanced diet also requires healthy fats. Healthy fats that help to lower bad cholesterol and lower the risk of heart disease include the unsaturated fats found in foods like avocado and olive oil.

Vitamins and Minerals

In order to maintain optimal physiological function, a balanced diet should also include a variety of vitamins and minerals. Usually, these important minerals and vitamins are abundant in natural, whole foods. A high-quality multivitamin that is based on food can make up for any nutritional deficits, but it shouldn't be used in place of real, unprocessed foods.

Water

Water is necessary for proper digestion and toxin removal. By keeping muscles toned and limiting eating, it aids in maintaining a healthy weight. It is advised to consume 8 to 10 glasses daily.

In summary, achieving and sustaining a healthy weight requires keeping a balanced diet. Eating a range of nutrient-dense foods, such as lean proteins, complex carbohydrates, healthy fats, and drinking plenty of water will help you lose weight and keep your health at its best.

Managing Food Cravings

For many individuals attempting to reduce weight, food cravings are a regular issue. Cravings not only make it challenging to avoid unhealthy foods and snacks, but they can also frequently result in overeating. Thankfully, there are ways to control food cravings and maintain a weight loss plan.

Identification is the first step in controlling food urges. Are there any particular meals that you frequently crave? Maybe some cookies or a certain kind of candy? Cravings are typically linked to emotional eating, which is the propensity to eat unhealthy foods to deal with stress, unpleasant feelings, or boredom. It will be simpler to develop a disciplined strategy to control your impulses if you have identified the foods and circumstances that lead to food cravings.

Practise mindful eating as one of the most crucial measures. Instead than eating aimlessly in front of the TV or computer, concentrate on taking pleasure in each mouthful of your meal. By allotting some time to sit down, unwind, and pay attention to your meal, you may practise being attentive. Eat slowly, savour the flavour of what you're eating, and express gratitude for it.

Another method for controlling food cravings is to prepare meals and snacks a few days in advance. Make a menu that features wholesome foods like fruits, vegetables, whole grains, lean proteins, and healthy fats. Organising your meals in advance and making sure you have wholesome foods on hand for when cravings occur can also be beneficial.

It's also critical to control your stress and get enough sleep. Getting enough sleep can control your hormones and lessen the need to eat in order to feel better. Deep breathing, meditation, and yoga are just a few strategies for reducing stress.

Finally, if you succumb to temptation, try not to be too hard on yourself. Everyone makes mistakes occasionally, so don't be hard on yourself if you do. Instead, concentrate on staying the course the bulk of the time and take use of your mistakes to improve.

It is feasible to effectively manage food cravings and maintain a weight-loss plan by recognizing urges, making preparations, eating mindfully, managing stress, and developing excellent sleep habits. Your health and wellness objectives may be achievable with some effort and practice.

Time Management Tips

It takes an extraordinary level of commitment and self-control to lose weight. To achieve your goals, you must learn to effectively manage your time in addition to carefully monitoring your food and engaging in regular exercise. Any weight loss programme must include time management. Maintaining focus can be a difficult and stressful undertaking, but with the appropriate methods and advice, you can succeed.

The numerous time management strategies to make sure your weight loss programme is successful are covered in the next section.

1. Plan Ahead

The most important tip for efficient time management is to prepare ahead. After defining realistic goals, make a schedule that will help you reach them. By doing this, you can keep structured and on schedule.

Make a schedule detailing what needs to be done when. Prioritise projects based on their relevance and break up huge jobs into manageable chunks. Reminders can help you keep on track by ensuring that you remember them.

2. Prioritize

Setting priorities for your jobs is essential if you want to maximise your time. Choose the tasks that are most important to you and concentrate on them. You'll be able to stay on track and use your time more effectively as a result.

Understand when to refuse. You will occasionally need to select between chores, so set priorities and make sure you are focusing on the most crucial things. You can maintain focus and direction by saying "no" to some chores.

3. Use Technology

Utilise the numerous technologies that are available. To help you stay on track, you may set up email and text reminders. You may maintain organisation and motivation by using internet tools and applications.

4. Manage Stress

Losing weight can be frustrating and challenging. Make sure your tension is being controlled. Regular exercise, yoga, and meditation can help you manage your stress and stick to your goals.

5. Prepare in Advance

When it comes to time management, preparation is essential. Plan your meals carefully, especially if you are on a special diet. Additionally, you can prepare meals or snacks in advance for the week so they are ready when you are.

6. Break It Up

By dividing your work into smaller tasks, you might be able to handle it better. Break up your workouts into shorter, more effective sessions as opposed to conducting one long one. This will help you stay motivated and on track

.7. Take Breaks

It's crucial to take breaks frequently during the day. Your energy levels and focus will stay high as a result. To guarantee that you are rested and prepared to face the day, make sure you are receiving enough sleep.

Any weight loss programme that is successful must have good time management. You may better manage your time and stay focused on achieving your goals by using the advice provided above. You can succeed if you use the appropriate tactics.

Incorporating Superfoods into Your Diet

Superfoods are foods that are very nutrient-dense and frequently brimming with minerals, vitamins, and antioxidants. They can aid in promoting weight loss, enhancing general health, and even lowering the risk of chronic illnesses like cancer and heart disease. Superfoods can be a terrific way to nourish your body and speed up your metabolism so that you can achieve your weight loss objectives.

You may incorporate a variety of superfoods into your regular diet, including dark leafy greens, nuts & seeds, berries, and whole grains. These superfoods contain all the vitamins, minerals, and other elements you require each day along with a wealth of antioxidants and nutrients that can help you feel satiated for longer. Look for foods that are high in protein, fibre, vitamins, and minerals while being low in calories and fat for weight loss.

Dark Leafy Greens: Leafy greens are highly nutrient dense and packed with antioxidants. Some examples of these greens include kale, spinach, rocket and collard greens. Additionally, they are high in fibre and low in calories. Consuming dark leafy greens regularly can assist to improve digestion and lower bodily inflammation. To receive the maximum benefit from these superfoods, use them into salads, smoothies, or even cooked meals.

Nuts and seeds are a fantastic source of protein, fibre, and good fats. They are also rich in nutrients and antioxidants. They can increase metabolism and help you feel fuller longer if you include them in your diet. For an added nutritional boost, you may use nuts and seeds into baked products, smoothies, yoghurt, and salads.

Berries: Due to their high antioxidant content, berries are superfoods that have a number of health advantages. Strawberries, blueberries, raspberries, and blackberries are all great providers of fibre, vitamins, and minerals. They can aid in reducing inflammation and enhancing general wellness. A cup of berries can be a terrific addition to your regular diet to help you get an extra burst of antioxidants.

Whole Grains: Whole grains are an important part of any healthy diet. They are packed with fiber and a variety of essential vitamins and minerals. Incorporating whole grains into your meal plan can help to improve your digestion, reduce hunger, and keep your energy levels up throughout the day. Look for whole grain breads, pastas, quinoa, and oats to get the most out of your meal plan.

Superfoods are a great method to increase metabolism, decrease appetite, and lower your chance of developing chronic diseases. To get the most out of your dieting efforts, make sure to incorporate a range of nutrient-rich meals into your daily meal plan. For optimum health and weight loss, include dark leafy greens, nuts and seeds, berries, and whole grains in your daily diet plan

.

Setting Achievable Goals for Weight Loss

The idea of achieving long-term outcomes when it comes to weight loss sometimes overwhelms and intimidates people. It's critical to keep in mind that losing weight is a process, not an overnight change. To lose weight in a way that is sustainable, you must be committed to a healthy lifestyle. Setting attainable goals will help you stay motivated and on course during your journey.

Any weight loss journey should start with setting a healthy goal. Setting an impossible goal is a common mistake that can result in frustration and a lack of progress. Setting reasonable expectations is crucial when choosing a healthy objective. Losing 10 pounds in a month may be an ambitious (and maybe risky) goal to set. Losing 5-7 pounds in a month is a far more realistic and sustainable objective.

It's crucial to divide bigger goals into smaller, more manageable ones. As they are more likely to be accomplished, these more manageable objectives could mean the difference between success and failure. For instance, if someone wants to lose 20 pounds, it's necessary to divide that objective into 4 manageable monthly weight loss targets of 5 pounds each. This will support the individual's motivation and progress throughout the entire procedure.

It's critical to keep in mind that development takes time and cannot be hastened while establishing realistic objectives for weight loss. In order to remain committed to one's goals, it is crucial to concentrate on the process rather than the outcomes. Additionally, it's crucial to recognise and appreciate tiny accomplishments along the way because they might support motivational growth.

While it might be challenging to remain committed and focused during a weight loss journey, one can do so by setting manageable goals along the route. Setting attainable goals might be essential to achieving long-term success because they offer structure and accountability to the process.

Staying Motivated for Weight Loss

There is no doubting the beneficial effects that good habits and weight loss can have on our general health and happiness. It's crucial to put in the effort and commitment required to make our diet and exercise objectives a reality if we want to look and feel our best. Unfortunately, this might feel like an uphill battle, and maintaining motivation to lose weight can be quite difficult depending on our current situation and lifestyle.

It's crucial to comprehend the significance of maintaining motivation, regardless of whether you're starting from scratch or have been having trouble achieving your goals. The likelihood of success actually decreases dramatically if you're not driven, even with the best diet and exercise regimen. This chapter will go into great detail on the value of maintaining motivation and how to do it in order to achieve your goals.

Making a consistent effort to follow healthy practises every day is the key to weight loss and good health. The process to losing weight involves a great deal of drive because eating well, exercising, and sticking to a plan are crucial components.

When you don't want to go to the gym or it's hard to resist late-night food, motivation helps you get through those tough times. Being highly driven makes it simpler to resist these temptations and stick with your plan. Additionally, motivation helps us continue through difficult activities and fosters resilience. For instance, motivation can keep us continuing when we encounter a challenging workout, observe slow progress, or don't receive the outcomes we'd hoped for. It can also serve as a reminder that with time and effort, we will succeed.

SONIA FLETCHER

The key to staying motivated is having a clear goal in mind. This means that you need to know exactly what your end goal is and be able to set realistic milestones along the way to build up to it. It also helps to have a plan and simple action steps that will help you to achieve your goal. For instance, if your goal is to run four times a week, you should make sure to plan out your runs and get a clear idea of how to fit them into your schedule.

Another suggestion is to keep track of your accomplishments and treat yourself. It's vital to reward yourself occasionally when you meet a goal, and keeping track of your weight and other measurements might assist to keep you motivated. You will be inspired to continue on your path by this.

Last but not least, keep in mind that there will be ups and downs. This is only a normal aspect of any travel, so it's crucial to maintain concentration and finally return your attention to your objectives.

A commitment to long-lasting, sustainable change is required to lose weight and get healthier. Keep a specific objective in mind, have a plan, and treat yourself to something enjoyable to help you become and stay motivated. Although it can be difficult to motivate oneself to lose weight, it is possible and the rewards are worthwhile.

Tips for Sticking to Your Plan

1. Develop a Long-Term Plan: Having a clearly defined target is the key to staying with any plan. Your strategy should be customised to meet your specific objectives and account for all relevant elements, such as

your present weight, dietary habits, lifestyle, and exercise routines. This will assist you in developing an achievable and realistic plan.

2. Establish Reasonable Goals: It's critical to establish goals that are both realistic and attainable. Make sure your objectives are realistic; if they are, it will be more difficult for you to follow through on your plan. Instead, break down your goals into manageable chunks so you can achieve each one and celebrate your accomplishments along the way.

3. Monitor Your Progress: Monitor your progress to ensure that you are moving in the proper direction. You'll be more motivated to stay on track if you track your progress. Make sure you are documenting your emotional and mental well-being in addition to your weight loss.

4. Celebrate Setbacks: There will be instances when you don't achieve your goal because success doesn't happen overnight. It's crucial to take time to enjoy your setbacks since they will teach you and make you stronger.

5. Be Kind To Yourself: If you don't achieve your goals, try not to be too hard on yourself. Do your best, and don't berate yourself for little slip-ups. Instead, concentrate on the good things and use these challenges to strengthen you.

6. Avoid Temptations: Resisting temptation is one of the hardest things to do when following a plan. Practise mindful eating to prevent this, and be careful to exercise self-control when it comes to urges. Making an environment free from temptations to deviate from your plan, such as

avoiding trigger foods or keeping an eye on your dieting spouse, can also be beneficial.

7. Keep Hydrated: Staying on track requires drinking enough of water. Water can help you feel satisfied for longer and can also help you stop craving certain foods. Keep yourself hydrated to help keep your energy levels up when exercising.

8. Start Exercising Gradually: Exercise is a crucial part of any weight loss strategy. As you get more fit, gradually up the intensity of your workouts from a low base. This will keep you motivated and make sure that your body isn't being overworked.

9. Find assistance: It might be challenging to stick to a plan, so it's critical to seek out assistance from individuals close to you. Having a conversation companion and someone who can relate may be really helpful, whether it's through dieting together or joining a weight reduction support group.

10. Reward Yourself: Giving yourself a reward for following your strategy might help you stay motivated and focused. Allow yourself to indulge in a small treat every now and again, or treat yourself to a shopping spree or massage when you accomplish a goal. This will make it easier for you to stick to your strategy and increase the fun of the journey to your goal.

Avoiding Weight Loss Plateaus

For many dieters, reaching a weight loss plateau can be very frustrating. A disappointed dieter could be tempted to give up since it frequently seems as though their efforts and dedication have been in vain and no progress has been made. But it is feasible to keep working towards your goal weight and avoid hitting a weight reduction plateau. The following advice will help you prevent weight loss plateaus:

1. Track Progress and Modify Calorie Intake: Tracking your progress and changing your calorie intake can help you avoid reaching a plateau. You may identify when a plateau is starting to set in by routinely checking your weight, writing down what you eat, calculating your portions, and evaluating your workout regimen, for example. This early notice offers you the chance to make the required adjustments, such changing your food or upping your exercise routine, to maintain your weight reduction programme.

2. Increase Your Exercise: You can overcome a weight loss stall by introducing new activities and stepping up your intensity. To effectively jump-start your metabolism, try including more strength training in your workouts along with increased cardio. You can get the metabolic boost you need to keep seeing improvements by intensifying your workout.

3. Consume More Protein: Consuming a diet high in protein is important for weight loss. In addition to aiding in muscle growth and repair, protein also takes longer to digest than other macronutrients, helping you feel filled for longer. Consuming adequate protein can also keep your metabolism running smoothly. For each kilogramme of body weight, try to consume 0.8–1.2 grammes of protein per day.

4. Adjust Your Meal Timings: Adjusting your meal schedule can assist in overcoming a plateau. Small, frequent snacks throughout the day can keep your metabolism humming and minimise motivation loss. Furthermore, having your final meal earlier in the day can aid in calorie burning during the night.

5. Consume Foods High in Fibre, Complex carbs, and Healthy Fats: Increasing your intake of foods high in fibre, complex carbs, and healthy fats can help you maintain a healthy metabolism. Fibre aids with digestion and helps you feel fuller for longer. You may provide your body a slow, consistent flow of energy by eating complex carbs like those found in fruits, vegetables, legumes, and whole grains. optimal fats are necessary for optimal bodily function and help keep your body full for hours. Some examples of these fats are those found in avocados, salmon, and almonds. Increased consumption of these meals can assist you in overcoming a weight loss plateau.

You should be well on your way to seeing results and avoiding a weight loss plateau if you stick to these suggestions. Keep your motivation up and your attention focused—you can do it!

Incorporating Physical Activity into Everyday Life

The idea of bringing physical activity into daily life can seem like a daunting effort in a world of hectic schedules. However, physical activity can and should be a significant part of a person's daily routine with a little bit of imagination, preparation, and work. Engagement requires an understanding of the value of physical activity for both improving physical health and its beneficial effects on psychological wellbeing.

Physical activity is crucial for enhancing or maintaining physical health, since it lowers the risk of obesity, cardiovascular disease, diabetes, some cancers, and diabetes-related complications. It also reduces stress, enhances mood and sleep quality, gives you more energy, and generally makes you feel better. Regular physical activity is crucial for achieving and preserving optimal health, according to research. The good news is that adding physical activity into daily life only needs a little amount of creative thought and planning; it does not require pricey gym subscriptions or dietary restrictions.

Physical activity can be incorporated into a daily schedule in a variety of ways. Examining the several simple ways that physical activity can be incorporated into daily life is crucial. Since everyone's everyday activities are diverse, they could call for various kinds of physical activity. Here are some illustrations of various forms of exercise:

•At Work - Aim to stand up and move about once every 30 to 60 minutes during the workday, or take little strolls at breaks. Additionally, wherever possible, think about using the stairs instead of the lift.

•At home - Try to get some exercise by going for a quick 10-minute walk, attending a yoga session, or doing some stretches instead of watching TV. Use nearby parks if they are available to get some fresh air, or get some small weights and resistance bands to work out at home.

•As a mode of transportation, try to bike or walk to work, school, chores or social events. This is not only stress-relieving but also good for the environment.

Incorporate exercise into your regular regimen. Setting aside time each day for exercise should be a top concern. Think about signing up for a fitness class, playing intramural sports, going for walks, or scheduling in an exercise class. Try to set reasonable objectives and enjoy yourself while exercising.

And finally, make exercise enjoyable. It can be made more pleasurable and motivating by incorporating it into a social situation, like a bike ride with friends or a game of frisbee in the park. Exercise with loved ones and friends can help foster positive connections, accountability, and drive.

In the end, including physical activity in daily activities is crucial for maintaining good mental, emotional, and physical health. There are always ways to incorporate physical activity into daily living, despite how busy life may be. Improved physical and mental health, as well as a healthier lifestyle, can result from developing and maintaining routines, appreciating the value of physical activity for health, and making it enjoyable.

Meal Planning for Busy Schedules

One of the best strategies to manage weight loss is to meal plan for hectic schedules. It's a quick and practical method to plan nutrient-balanced meals, make a shopping list, and stay under a set spending limit. Without spending hours in the kitchen, a thoughtful meal plan will help you ensure that you are eating a balanced diet and avoiding harmful options.

Meal planning begins with a lifestyle assessment. Spend some time considering your eating patterns and the kinds of things you frequently order at restaurants or buy at the grocery store. This can help you have a better sense of the things you should include in your meal plan.

It's time to start considering how to organise your meals after you have a clear notion of the kinds of foods you want to include in your meal plan. Create a weekly meal plan that you can adhere to on a daily basis to start. Throughout the week, make a note of the times you plan to have breakfast, lunch, supper, and snacks. Snacks should be a part of your strategy because they can assist prevent hunger throughout the day and offer more nutritionally balanced food.

Be sure to arrange a variety of meals while making your menu. Make sure to include a variety of proteins, fruits, vegetables, and complex carbohydrates in your meal plan. To avoid getting bored with your routine, you might also switch up your meals. Instead of using chicken or beef, experiment with substituting other proteins like fish, pig, or tofu.

Once your menu is finalised, you should make a shopping list. Note everything you require, including the precise quantities of each ingredient. This will make grocery shopping more effective and ensure that you have all the ingredients on hand when it's time to eat.

SONIA FLETCHER

Last but not least, remember to schedule cooking hours for each meal. When you have a hectic schedule, it might be difficult to find the time to prepare, so try to plan for quick and simple meals. Utilise quick cooking techniques like grilling, baking, and sautéing. Try setting aside time on the weekends to make a few dishes in advance if you require more hands-on time in the kitchen. You'll have wonderful, nutritious meals prepared in this manner to eat throughout the week.

A smart strategy to manage weight loss is to meal prepare for hectic schedules. Meal planning takes some practise to get into, but if you stick with it, you'll be able to eat better-for-you meals without putting in as much work. These suggestions will make it simple for you to put together a balanced, healthy food plan that fits your lifestyle.

PART IV: LIFESTYLE CHANGES

Finding Social Support

One of the most crucial elements of a successful weight loss journey can be social support. The difference between success and failure can often be determined by a person's ability to build a strong network of allies and supporters. Unfortunately, a lot of people struggle to find social assistance because they don't know where to look.

Reaching out to current relationships or even establishing new ones is one of the best places to start. You can turn to friends, family, and even coworkers for help and accountability. Talking to someone who can provide an unbiased viewpoint can be really helpful. Knowing that someone else is keeping track of our progress also encourages us to continue on course.

There are also innumerable online communities of people who are trying to lose weight, some of which were created by experts and others by people just like us. Joining one of these online groups, forums, or social media communities is a terrific opportunity to meet like-minded individuals who can provide support virtually and occasionally in person. Being able to lean on fellow members who have overcome similar obstacles and succeeded can be very motivating.

Additionally, a lot of gyms and health clubs provide group classes that foster social interaction. These programmes offer a terrific setting for meeting new people and discussing success because they are frequently targeted to certain goals, like weight loss. You may even come across neighbourhood clubs or organisations catering to a particular demographic, like elderly or female-only weight loss programmes.

In our daily lives, it's critical to actively seek out social support. Finding others who are also having difficulties with their weight loss objectives, whether in person or online, can be very beneficial. Success stories, queries, suggestions, and words of support can all come up in conversations. Making connections with people who have comparable difficulties can mean the difference between a weight reduction journey's success and failure.

.

Making Time for Yourself

When it comes to losing weight, time management is essential. To achieve your objective, you must set aside time to take care of your body and mind. You can stay on track with your weight-loss objectives and increase your chances of success by learning how to prioritise the various facets of your life. Here are some ideas to help you prioritise your well-being and maintain your attention on your weight-loss goals.

Start by setting reasonable expectations for the amount of time you can devote to exercising and taking care of yourself. Consider how much time you can devote to exercise realistically each day or each week, as well as how much time you can set out for leisure or self-care activities. Once you've made a plan, follow it.

Establish a sustainable habit that you can adhere to as a part of making time for yourself. Establish a balanced schedule that allows for time for physical activity, a nutritious diet, and rest and relaxation.

Make self-care a priority. Doing self-care activities can help you stay motivated and on track with your weight loss objectives. Think about engaging in stress-relieving hobbies like yoga, meditation, proper sleep, music listening, reading, or any other activity.

Establish a "me" day by setting aside at least one day each week for activities that are exclusively for you. Without having to worry about any plans or obligations, spend the day relaxing or engaging in something you enjoy.

Utilise technology: It may be a fantastic tool for helping you manage your time and stay focused on your objectives. Use apps to keep track of your workout progress, set alarms to remind you to eat well or spend a few minutes in yoga or meditation, and wear fitness trackers to keep track of your steps and hold yourself responsible.

Find an accountability partner: Making time for yourself and maintaining your success can be made much easier by working with an accountability partner who can keep you motivated and on track with your goals. It might be a member of your family, a close friend, or a personal trainer who can keep you motivated and focused.

Creating time for oneself is crucial if you want to lose weight. Your hard work will pay off if you take the time to establish a balanced routine, give self-care activities top priority, and make the most of technology. You can quickly accomplish your goals if you put some effort and time into it.

Preventing Binge Eating

One of the most prevalent eating disorders is binge eating, which can have negative health effects. To preserve excellent physical and emotional health, it's critical to learn how to identify and prevent it.

Periods of excessive eating, or "bingeing," are the hallmark of the eating disorder known as binge eating disorder (BED), which is then followed by feelings of guilt, shame, or melancholy. Contrary to people with bulimia nervosa, those with BED do not purge or engage in excessive activity to make up for their overeating. No matter their age, gender, or body type, anyone can experience binge eating, however those who are overweight or obese are more prone to do so.

As well as frequent post-eating feelings of guilt, shame, or sorrow, episodes of devouring great amounts of food quickly (sometimes all in one day) are the hallmarks of binge eating. Other signs include eating till you feel uncomfortable, eating even when you're not hungry, eating in front of others, and feeling like you can't stop eating even when you're full.

Although the precise origins of binge eating are unknown, a variety of biological, psychological, and social factors are likely to be involved. Hormonal imbalances and ongoing stress are examples of biological causes, whereas emotional eating and self-esteem issues are examples of psychological ones. Environmental triggers, such holidays or the availability of certain meals, as well as cultural influences, like viewpoints on body size or body image, can all be considered social causes.

THere are some steps you can take to stop or cut back on binge eating episodes.

1. Healthy Eating - The first step in preventing binges is to eat a balanced, wholesome diet. Small, regular meals can assist maintain stable blood sugar levels and stave off hunger pangs throughout the day.

2. Manage Portion Sizes - Eating smaller meals more regularly, as opposed to one large meal, can be good. By doing this, you can prevent overeating and guarantee that you obtain enough nourishment throughout the day..

3. Avoid Trigger Foods - It's crucial to your health to recognise and stay away from "trigger" foods that might cause binges. This can include junk food, sugary snacks, and anything else that is deemed to be particularly unhealthy or bad for you.

4. Recognise Emotional Triggers - Emotional eating frequently leads to binge eating, so it's important to learn good coping mechanisms. This can entail doing stress-relieving things like exercising, writing in a notebook, talking to a reliable friend, or journaling.

5. Seek specialised help - If binge eating is a problem for you, it's imperative that you seek specialised help. With the assistance of a doctor or mental health professional, you can identify the underlying causes of binge eating and develop coping mechanisms.

SONIA FLETCHER

occurrence is feasible to preserve good physical and emotional health by being aware of the warning symptoms and risk factors of binge eating and implementing preventive actions to lower the likelihood of occurrence.

Understanding Mental Health and Wellness

Two of the most crucial aspects of reaching effective, long-term weight loss objectives are mental health and wellness. When people are focused on achieving their weight reduction goals, the significance of comprehending and managing mental health and wellness is sometimes disregarded, despite the fact that this is an essential step in the procedure.

We must first take into account how intimately linked mental health and wellness are. Our ability to function emotionally, cognitively, and behaviorally is linked to our mental health. A state of being physically, mentally, and emotionally healthy is referred to as wellness. Since mental health has a big impact on our general health and wellness, mental health and wellness are closely related.

The foundation of mental health and wellness is a strong sense of self-worth and confidence. Strong self-esteem and confidence are frequently linked to a higher propensity to make healthier decisions and more success in losing weight. In the absence of these skills, people may be more prone to use compulsive or emotional eating as a coping strategy for negative thoughts or feelings and less likely to exercise regularly and make healthy dietary changes that might encourage long-term success.

Along with self-esteem, managing stress and emotional suffering is an essential component of mental health and wellness. Making the consistent lifestyle changes necessary for weight loss might be difficult when under stress since it can be difficult to focus and think properly. Furthermore, engaging in stress-reduction practises like yoga, mindfulness, and relaxation methods may inspire people to adopt wiser food and activity choices and reduce emotional eating.

Last but not least, creating a supportive and happy environment is crucial for achieving and sustaining excellent mental health. Making connections with peers, family, and friends can make people feel less alone and more supported during their weight reduction journey. For many people, participating in support groups or online communities can be extremely beneficial.

In general, successful and long-lasting weight loss and enhanced physical and emotional wellbeing depend on having a solid understanding of mental health and wellness. Increased self-esteem and self-care practises, an improved stress response, and a more uplifting and encouraging social network can all be results of good mental health and wellness. Gaining these abilities can be advantageous for long-term weight loss success and have a good impact on general health and wellness.

Improving Body Image and Self-Esteem

Body image and self-esteem are closely linked. A person with low self-esteem may be uncomfortable with how they look and have a bad relationship with food, which can result in unhealthful weight increase and a dissatisfaction with their body shape. Just as physical unhappiness can lead to low self-esteem and poor mental health. At least 30 million Americans of all ages suffer from an eating disorder, and roughly 20 million women and 10 million men encounter an eating disorder that is clinically serious at some point in their lives, according to the National Eating Disorders Association. It goes without saying that significant issues with body image and self-esteem can and frequently do result in disordered eating. Therefore, it is essential for both successful weight loss and maintenance to have a positive body image and feel good about yourself.

In today's society, media messages can establish an unattainable standard for beauty, which can result in low self-esteem and feelings of inadequacy. The "ideal" body image is one where a person is skinny, tall, and generally attractive. This body image is promoted by magazines, television, movies, and other visual media. This ideal is frequently difficult or impossible to attain, and those who are unable to do so may experience body dissatisfaction. Research has also shown that media messages can affect how people behave when it comes to food; when exposed to pictures of skinny models, people often consume smaller amounts of food or skip meals entirely.

There are a number of ways to help someone combat the impact of media messages that might lead to low self-esteem and a negative body image. Avoiding periodicals, TV shows, and other media that promote feelings of inadequacy or negative body image is crucial for limiting exposure to media messaging. Finding real-life positive role models who provide an alternative to unrealistic beauty standards, such as friends, family, or mentors, is also beneficial.

By substituting unfavourable attitudes with more sensible approaches to one's body, those who struggle with low self-esteem owing to body size or shape can also develop a positive self-image. People can learn to focus on healthy behaviours like exercise, a balanced diet, and mindful eating rather than their size or weight. People can also take care of themselves by doing things like yoga, getting proper sleep, and using other relaxing methods.

In conclusion, it's critical to understand how media messages affect one's self-esteem and body image and to actively combat harmful messages. The techniques described in this chapter can assist people in developing a more positive relationship with their bodies. Improving body image and self-esteem requires time and patience. People can take charge of their health and wellness, experience the advantages of successful weight loss and maintenance, and take control of their relationship with food by developing a healthier self-image.

Setting Long-Term Goals and Strategies

It need both short-term and long-term tactics to lose weight. Effective short-term tactics are crucial for quick outcomes, but long-term plans are required for results that will last and be permanent. Anyone wishing to attain and maintain long-term success in their weight loss journey must set long-term goals and methods. For those trying to move in the direction of a healthy lifestyle, this chapter will offer guidance on how to develop long-term objectives and plans.

Long-term objectives and plans are crucial for weight loss because they promote a change in lifestyle. While short-term tactics like calorie restriction or increased exercise can produce noticeable effects quickly, these tactics are frequently unsustainable. Long-term objectives and plans demand more work and dedication, but they can produce results that stay longer. Long-term objectives and strategies make it more likely that the person will be able to change their way of life for the better and permanently.

Long-term objectives should be both attainable and practical. Aiming high is crucial, but it's also necessary to make realistic goals that you can accomplish with commitment and effort. A person trying to shed 50 pounds, for instance, shouldn't aim to do so in a single month. Such an objective is unattainable and would almost certainly result in disappointment and frustration. Instead, they ought to make more manageable, gradual progress, like reducing 5 pounds each month.

Setting both short-term and long-term goals is crucial. These objectives have to be adaptable and modified in light of the person's development. If a person wants to lose 50 pounds, they can start with a 10-pound goal and then establish new ones each month as the weight is shed.

Long-term objectives must also be quantifiable. For the person to gauge how well they are doing, there should be a means to track development. This could involve activities like regularly weighing oneself or taking weekly or monthly measurements. This will enable them to monitor their progress and keep them motivated.

It's critical to create and put into action long-term plans that will help the person achieve their objectives. These tactics could involve food adjustments, increased physical activity, and behavioural adjustments.

It's crucial to create a healthy eating strategy that incorporates whole grains, lean proteins, fresh fruits and vegetables, and healthy fats. Limiting added sugars and processed foods should also be a component of the strategy. An effective food plan can be developed and followed with the help of a nutritionist.

It's crucial to up your physical activity if you want to modify your lifestyle. Depending on the individual's degree of fitness, they might need to start out gently. For a newbie, beginning a walking programme might be an excellent place to start. The intensity and duration of the activity can be gradually increased as the person advances.

SONIA FLETCHER

Finally, it's crucial to concentrate on changing your behaviour. This can involve creating a brand-new daily routine that emphasises healthful behaviours like drinking more water, making meals in advance, and getting enough sleep. By concentrating on these actions, a new, healthy lifestyle can be developed.

Anyone wishing to advance in their weight loss journey must establish long-term goals and plans. Making a plan that includes healthier food, more exercise, and behavioural changes is necessary for achieving long-term success. Setting reasonable and achievable goals is vital. Long-term objectives and plans can aid in making lasting changes and ensuring successful and long-lasting results with commitment and hard work.

PART V: OTHER CONSIDERATIONS

Dealing with Food Allergies

It might be challenging to keep up a healthy weight and way of life if you have food allergies. More than 12 million Americans suffer from food allergies, which can have both immediate and long-term negative health effects. Weight loss might be easier to maintain if you are aware of the steps you can take to manage food allergies.

Start by Identifying Food Allergies

Finding out what foods you are allergic to is the first and most crucial step in controlling your allergies. Food allergies to milk, eggs, peanuts, tree nuts, wheat, soy, fish, and shellfish are among the most prevalent.

These reactions might be modest, like feeling a little sick after eating something, or severe, like anaphylaxis.

For a formal diagnosis of any food allergies you feel may exist, consult your healthcare professional. The healthcare professional might advise performing an allergic skin test, eating a tiny "challenge" amount of the suspected culprits, or following an elimination diet.

Making Dietary Adjustments

You can modify your diet after you have a better grasp of potential food allergens. You might need to restrict or stay away from a few substances to prevent an allergic response. Your healthcare practitioner can offer alternatives and a list of foods that are safe to eat.

Educate Yourself

Learning how to identify the signs of an allergic reaction is one of the most crucial steps in controlling food allergies. Hives, itching, swelling of the eyes, face, throat, or tongue, difficulty breathing, dizziness, lightheadedness, or chest pain are typical symptoms of an allergic reaction. For weight loss to be successful, it's essential to learn to recognise these symptoms.

It's also crucial to develop your ability to properly read menus and food labels. Learn about the components of any products you might be considering consuming. Always let the restaurant know if you have any allergies.

Stay Prepared

Anaphylaxis can sometimes be brought on by exposure to the dietary allergen. It's critical to constantly be ready for emergencies. Your doctor will suggest a strategy that involves keeping an epinephrine auto-injector on hand in case of an emergency.

Although managing food allergies might be challenging, it is doable if you know how. You may maintain a healthy lifestyle and, ultimately, a healthy weight, by following these instructions.

Managing Polycystic Ovarian Syndrome

Controlling the symptoms and averting long-term problems are the main objectives of PCOS management. Menstrual irregularities, weight gain, excessive hair growth, acne, and infertility are all common signs of PCOS. Chronic PCOS can lead to long-term health issues like diabetes, hypertension, heart disease, and endometrial cancer. To effectively manage PCOS, it's crucial to engage with a healthcare professional to create a personalised treatment plan.

Losing weight is important for managing PCOS. Being overweight may make PCOS symptoms worse, making management more difficult. The symptoms of acne, excessive hair growth, and irregular periods can all be alleviated by losing weight. Furthermore, it can reduce the likelihood of long-term conditions including diabetes and heart disease. For weight loss, it's essential to keep up a nutritious diet with a well-balanced mix of protein, fruits, vegetables, and complete grains. A weight-loss plan also needs to incorporate regular exercise.

The usage of prescription drugs is a crucial component of managing PCOS. Oral contraceptives and anti-androgens, for example, can help regulate menstrual cycles and lessen symptoms like excessive hair growth and acne. In some circumstances, PCOS-affected women may be given reproductive drugs to aid in conception. To assist control blood sugar levels, doctors may prescribe insulin-lowering drugs if necessary. It's crucial to schedule routine appointments with a doctor in order to track the effectiveness of prescription drugs and modify treatment as necessary.

Changes in lifestyle are also crucial for managing PCOS. Yoga, meditation, and other stress-reduction practises can help lower stress levels and insulin levels. Stress can be decreased by getting enough sleep and managing your time well. Additionally, avoiding smoking and abusing alcohol can lower your risk of developing long-term health issues.

If PCOS symptoms are present, it's critical to consult a medical professional so that a customised management strategy may be created. With the assistance of a medical professional, lifestyle modifications and medications can be utilised to manage symptoms and lower the possibility of long-term health consequences. One of the most crucial elements in managing PCOS is weight loss because it can lessen symptoms and the chance of long-term health effects. To fully benefit from weight loss, a balanced diet and regular physical activity are essential.

Managing Endometriosis

Endometriosis can seriously impact a woman's life and is a crippling, misdiagnosed ailment. Endometriosis is thought to afflict up to 10% of women in the United States, but given the stigma associated with the disease and the lack of knowledge around it, the actual percentage is probably much higher.

The challenge of managing weight loss is particularly difficult for women with endometriosis. Widespread pain and inflammation brought on by endometriosis can result in changes in appetite, exhaustion, and decreased physical activity. This can lead to weight gain and a higher risk of metabolic diseases like diabetes, hypertension, and high cholesterol.

It's critical to comprehend how endometriosis and weight loss are related in order to manage the condition successfully. Severe abdominal pain brought on by endometriosis might make it difficult to follow diets and exercise routines. An endometriosis patient should therefore concentrate on establishing realistic, doable activity and dietary goals.

In order to manage endometriosis, one must concentrate on making appropriate food choices. A diet rich in nutrients, nutritionally balanced, and emphasising whole grains, fresh produce, healthy fats, and lean protein is crucial. Consuming a lot of fiber-rich foods can help to reduce inflammation and promote healthy digestion, both of which can improve mood and general well-being.

SONIA FLETCHER

Losing weight and controlling endometriosis both need exercise. Walking, riding, swimming, and hiking are all examples of cardiovascular exercises that can assist to reduce inflammation and promote overall wellness. Additionally, strength training is crucial since it can increase strength and endurance.

Stress management is essential for treating endometriosis and weight reduction in addition to diet and exercise. Inflammation can be directly impacted by stress, which can also make endometriosis symptoms worse. Yoga, meditation, and tai chi are examples of mind-body practises that can be helpful in lowering stress.

Finally, it's crucial to discuss any dietary or lifestyle adjustments being made with a doctor in order to manage endometriosis and weight loss. Given the complexity of endometriosis, it's critical to ensure that the patient is receiving the proper care and support from their physician.

In conclusion, managing the relationship between endometriosis and weight loss might be challenging. Endometriosis and weight loss can be successfully managed by concentrating on food, exercise, stress management, and listening to medical guidance.

.

SONIA FLETCHER

Understanding Thyroid Dysfunction

The term "thyroid dysfunction" is used to describe a variety of thyroid conditions, including hypothyroidism and hyperthyroidism. The thyroid gland produces and releases hormones that are essential for the body's metabolism, the generation of energy, and general health in both circumstances. Up to 20 million Americans are thought to be affected by thyroid disorders, with women five to eight times more likely than males to be affected.

Understanding Anyone seeking to lose weight must address thyroid dysfunction. The body's metabolic rate and the pace at which calories are expended are determined by the T3 and T4 hormones, which are generated by the thyroid gland. A surplus of calories may be stored as fat when these hormone levels are out of balance, which can result in weight gain and make it challenging to decrease weight.

The most prevalent thyroid ailment, hypothyroidism, or an underactive thyroid, causes a decrease in thyroid hormone production. Increased tiredness, dry skin, constipation, memory problems, depression, and weight gain are all signs of hypothyroidism. Hypothyroidism can cause major health problems like heart disease, infertility, or stroke if it is not treated.

When the thyroid gland generates excessive amounts of the hormones T3 and T4, hyperthyroidism, or an overactive thyroid, can result. Weight loss, a faster heartbeat, sweating, anxiety and uneasiness, diarrhoea, and tremors are all signs of hyperthyroidism. Hyperthyroidism can cause major health problems such an enlarged thyroid, an irregular heartbeat, and even death if it is not addressed.

The hormones generated by the thyroid gland play a significant role in controlling mood, emotional stability, and cognitive function in addition to the physical symptoms of thyroid diseases. Low thyroid hormone levels can cause irritability, forgetfulness, mood changes, anxiety, and sadness.

Accurately diagnosing the underlying reason is essential to treating thyroid disease. If the thyroid is producing too many or too few thyroid hormones, a quick blood test might help identify the problem. Treatment options include changing one's lifestyle, using medications, or perhaps even having surgery after the underlying reason has been determined.

People with thyroid dysfunction are frequently advised to make lifestyle changes because doing so can aid with overall health improvement. Better thyroid function and weight loss can be encouraged by following a nutritious diet, exercising frequently, controlling stress, and getting adequate sleep.

In conclusion, everyone trying to lose weight must comprehend thyroid dysfunction. A decrease in metabolic rate brought on by insufficient thyroid hormone synthesis might result in an excess of calories being stored as fat, whereas an increase in metabolic rate brought on by excessive thyroid hormone production can result in weight loss. Therefore, controlling and enhancing weight loss requires recognising and treating the underlying thyroid issue.

Eating with Diabetes

Many people find it challenging to eat while having diabetes. To maintain stable blood sugar levels while managing your diabetes, it's important to balance your meals' carbohydrate and protein intake. Every food group should be represented in a diabetes meal plan, including fruits, vegetables, lean meats, complete grains, and some dairy. The diabetes diet focuses on regulating when, what, and how much you eat.

Portion control is the most crucial element of eating when it comes to diabetes. The My Plate approach is one technique to guarantee that you are consuming the proper amount of food. You should do this by covering half of your plate with vegetables, one-fourth with a lean protein source, one-fourth with a complex carbohydrate, and finishing with a glass of low-fat milk or yoghurt. This will enable you to include the appropriate variety of meals at each meal. It is recommended to consume carbs from low glycemic index sources such whole grains, legumes, and starchy vegetables for people who need to limit their sugar intake.

For treating diabetes, it's also crucial to include healthy fats in the diet. Healthy fats, such those in nuts, avocados, olive oil, nuts, and olives, can aid in reducing the rate at which sugar is absorbed. The body needs healthy fats as fuel, and they can help us feel satisfied for extended periods of time.

It's crucial to consider portion amounts when eating snacks. Choose snacks that will give you both carbohydrates and protein, like hummus with veggies, nuts, or a piece of fruit with peanut butter, instead of sugary ones like candies or sugary cereal bars.

However, with a little mindfulness and knowledge of the foods that are ideal for your diabetes management, you can create a meal plan that is both healthy and fulfilling. Eating with diabetes does involve some forethought. You can manage your diabetes, maintain excellent health, and even support weight loss objectives by eating the proper balance of meals and closely monitoring your blood sugar levels.

The Aftermath of Weight Loss Surgery

Weight loss surgery is a major decision and one that should not be taken lightly. It involves many risks as well as potential benefits and can have a tremendous impact on an individual's health and lifestyle. Like any major medical decision, careful consideration should be given to the potential risks and rewards before making a decision.

Having weight loss surgery can have both physical and emotional side effects. Although weight reduction surgery can result in significant weight loss and a drop in BMI, there are a number of unfavourable side effects that can arise. Due to the significant alteration in their bodies and probable surgical complications, many patients report discomfort in the weeks after the treatment. Along with physical difficulties, people may experience mental and emotional difficulties as they become used to their new body types. It's crucial to go slowly and be kind to yourself during this stage because it can be disconcerting to go through such a rapid change.

On the plus side, weight loss surgery can have a significant and long-lasting impact on a person's health. Large, long-term weight loss has a number of possible health advantages, including reduced blood pressure, lowered cholesterol, and enhanced general health and wellbeing. Many patients also say they feel more energised and in better physical shape.

It is important to make a thoughtful decision about your life and health before having weight loss surgery. The technique has a lot of possible advantages and disadvantages, which people should carefully weigh before deciding to pursue it. It's critical for anyone thinking about surgery to be aware of any potential medical and psychological difficulties that can arise afterward. People can anticipate and handle any difficulties that arise during the process and perhaps reap the benefits of a healthier and happier life with the correct planning and assistance.

Working with A Dietician

Working with a dietitian is essential for achieving weight loss success. When it comes to nutrition, food, and exercise, a skilled dietician may offer priceless knowledge and experience that can help you achieve your goals.

A dietitian will consider your lifestyle, family history, and medical history as you work with them. Any probable medical issues or difficulties that might be keeping you from reducing weight are identified. With the use of this data, they design a diet strategy unique to your body.

You'll learn from the dietitian how to put together wholesome meals that are suitable for your requirements. They will discuss how crucial it is to consume all of the necessary nutrients found in food. Most dieticians will also educate you how to regulate your portion sizes.

You can get assistance from the dietitian with meal planning and food preparation. They can offer suggestions on what to put in your pantry and what vegetables to buy. Additionally, they can offer recipes and healthy snack ideas. They are a fantastic source of knowledge for tips on eating out healthily.

Your dietician can assist you in integrating your dietary plan into your daily routine once it has been created. They will talk about physical activity and make fitness recommendations to assist you in achieving your weight loss objectives.

They frequently provide suggestions, such as signing up for a certain workout class or joining a gym. They might also advise you to practise mindfulness or breathing techniques, particularly if stress is a problem for you.

There is no quick remedy for weight loss other than working with a dietitian. You and your dietitian will need to put some effort and time into the procedure. To attain your goals, you must be devoted to making the required adjustments.

If you ever feel unmotivated, your dietician can also provide you with support and advice. They can aid in goal-setting and offer you support

SONIA FLETCHER

when you falter. They are there to support you in staying on course and in enjoying your accomplishments.

Working with a dietitian is a terrific place to start if you feel like you need a little additional assistance with your weight loss quest. To assist you in achieving your objectives, a dietician can offer priceless expertise and encouragement.

Conclusion

In conclusion, Weight Loss for Women is an invaluable resource for anyone looking to make positive changes in their diet and lifestyle. It provides helpful tips on how to achieve realistic and sustainable weight loss goals, focusing on healthy eating habits, physical activity, and an overall balanced lifestyle. With this book as your guide, you can finally take control of your weight and health while avoiding unhealthy and extreme diets. Armed with the practical knowledge and tools outlined in this book, you can start down the path to a healthier you.